I0791295

ABOUT US

Lindsay

Although I was not what most would consider an athlete, Fitness has always been apart of my life. I was in gymnastics, dance, played volleyball and got my first Gold's gym membership at 17 years old. But it wasn't until college that I made fitness a priority!! I went from active high schooler who like the treadmill to hiring a personal trainer who actually showed me how to use the other things in the gym. It became an addiction and I never looked back. It wasn't, however, until after my second son was born that I took my fitness to another level. It wasn't enough anymore to do some light strength training a hours of cardio to lose weight I had to make changes to my diet and my workout routines. In an attempt to better educate myself I decided I would I get NASM certified as a personal trainer just for fun. Little did I know that my hobby would turn into this dream career. As a personal trainer it is my mission to not only transform and educate you, but to empower you and unleash your inner badass !!

Dizzy

As as kid I was pretty overweight and it had an affect on me. All the cool kids were the athletes and actually enjoyed time on the playground and I...well, wasn't. I enjoyed all the nerdy things but one of them was pro wrestling. As a teenager I decided I wanted to actually become one. But I needed to look like one! That is when a childhood friend taught me the art of bodybuilding. I finally learned that your body is totally in your control. Once I figured out the mysteries of the human body I needed to make sure no one around me was in the dark again! In 2014 I became a NASM Certified Personal Trainer and never looked back from fitness through all of my various lifestyle changes.

Mostly Fit

We started Mostly Fit as a podcast about the struggle between really really enjoys tacos and Dizzy has a slight enough people with the all-or-nothing attitude and everyone's life. We believe that everyone should be while still enjoying nights out from time to time majority of people are NOT professional thing around a pretty busy life. From day jobs need to be shredded, just Mostly Fit.

wanting to look good naked and treating yourself! Lindsay addiction to peanut butter. The fitness industry has unrealistic physique expectations, but that's not allowed to feel comfortable in his or her own skin without feeling guilty. We also realize that the athletes and we have to fit this entire fitness to kids to enjoying a glass of wine, we don't

MACROS

Proteins

Commonly referred to as the "building blocks of life," proteins are what the majority of what your body is made of. Proteins (which are made of smaller blocks called amino acids) make everything from your muscles to hair, skin, nails, and organ tissues! Some of the necessary amino acids can be produced by the human body but some, called "essential amino acids" must be taken in from food sources. We'll spare you all the complicated names, but just know that you need to eat protein to have a healthy and complete amino profile in your body.

When doing exercise, you create small micro tears in your muscle fibers that must be repaired. To aid in this repair, consuming protein is necessary. Think of your muscles similar to the way a rope is made—many tiny fibers that work together to form a larger, stronger unit.

Carbohydrates

"But I'm not supposed to eat carbs if I want to lose weight right?" WRONG! Carbohydrates are the number one energy source for the human body. To get sciencey for a moment, larger particles of carbohydrates called "starches" are broken down into simpler sugars to be burned off as energy. Only in a state of ketosis does your body use fat as a primary energy source.

Your body would actually rather use protein as energy before fat in the absence of carbs because fat has more than double the caloric value of protein (more on that later). Imagine if you had a $100 bill and a few $20 bills. It would be much easier to spend the 20's little by little because you know there is more value in the single 100. Your body was designed for optimum survival, so you kind of have to work with it. Eat your carbs so you feel better, perform better, and your friends like you better!

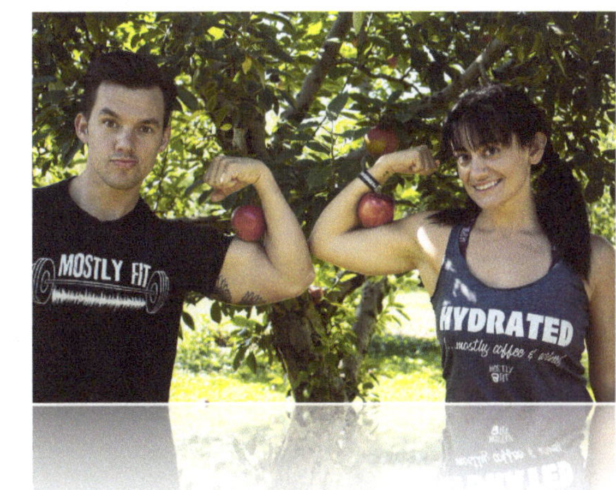

Fats

At this point, don't worry about what is a good fat and a bad fat. Let's just get into what fat is and why you need it. Obviously we store fat on our bodies and theoretically that should handle it right? Not so much, actually. The stored fat on your body is extra. Think about a squirrel in the winter who stores up food when it is in abundance just in case there won't be enough later. The squirrel doesn't mind if there's too much now, and neither does your body. Once it is stored, it is no longer used the same way as dietary fat.

On top of excess calorie storage, fat creates the membranes around cells, lubricates your blood vessels, and helps keep your hormones in line! Keeping a healthy balance of fat in the diet will keep your hair and skin looking nice as well as making your meals more satisfying (and tasty).

Water

An average adult is about 50-65% water. It makes up a majority of each part of your body and your muscles themselves are about 79% percent water! If you are exercising in any way your performance and recovery will benefit from getting an adequate water intake. Your blood is also mainly water so being hydrated allows all of the vitamins and minerals to be transported to their proper placement in the body as well. Other benefits of drinking water include better digestion, flushing out all of those mysterious toxins from the body, and keeping your skin hydrated as well. The best part about water is that it is FREE!

Alcohol

You didn't think we'd avoid this did you? No way! Just because alcohol isn't on the regular list doesn't mean that it is not a macronutrient. In short, alcohol is created from the fermentation of carbohydrates. After the process, the molecules are almost twice the caloric value (more on that later) so they should definitely be counted if you are trying to change or maintain a fit healthy body.

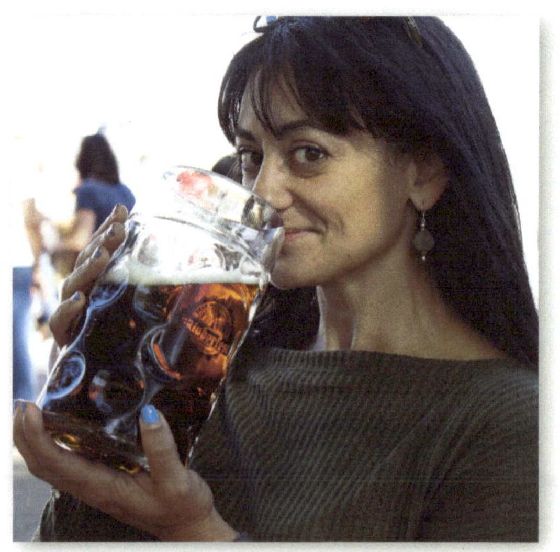

The downside to alcohol, though, is that your body registers it as a poison. It has to be metabolized first. As we said before, it has a caloric value, but no nutrition. If you have alcohol and food, and you exceed your daily caloric usage all the extra calories from food get stored as fat—and you have a hangover! (Hangovers are just dehydration and nutrient deficiencies.)

NUTRITION LABELS

Why Should I Care?

Nutrition labels seem to be one of the most ignored signs in the grocery store but they are among the most important things to learn when it comes to health and fitness. The image to the right is taken from a jar of peanut butter (of course) and is a prime example of the type of information that should be noticed.

What Is All This?

Firstly, you should take notice of the calories because that is the sum total of the macronutrients within this particular food. Whole food sources should be generally easiest to break down and categorize for which type of macro they might represent. The largest number should be the way you consider using a given food in your diet, based on your individual needs. As you see here, peanut butter's largest number is in fat at 16g while carbohydrates and protein are present in much lower numbers.

% Daily Value

Notice the "Percent Daily Value" has a star next to it, indicating at the bottom of the label that this number is based on a 2000 calorie diet. Everyone's individual dietary needs are different but this number was created based on the average American requirement to remain healthy.

Nutrition Facts

Serving Size 2 Tbsp (32g)
Servings Per Container About 23

Amount Per Serving

Calories 190   Calories from Fat 140

		% Daily Value*
Total Fat 16g		**25**%
Saturated Fat 3.5g		**18**%
Trans Fat 0g		
Cholesterol 0mg		**0**%
Sodium 150mg		**6**%
Total Carbohydrate 6g		**2**%
Dietary Fiber 2g		**8**%
Sugars 3g		
Protein 7g		

Vitamin A	0%	• Vitamin C	0%
Calcium	0%	• Iron	4%
Vitamin E	10%	• Niacin	20%

* Percent Daily Values are based on 2,000 calorie diet.

Other Information

Other information such as sodium, vitamins, and minerals are listed but their needs are entirely individual based on the types of foods you consume, the type of activities you do, and genetics. For instance, a person who works in a factory and spends most of the day sweating is going to have a greater need for sodium than a person of the same size and sex who works a desk job. To find exact needs, it is best to get blood work done at a clinic to read true levels and address micronutrient needs.

Serving Size

One of the absolute most important pieces of information on this label is the serving size. Many people ignore that portion all together and end up misreporting the calories they consume, and wonder why their bodies aren't changing. Knowledge is power and knowing how much you are eating could be a major factor in taking control of your health and fitness.

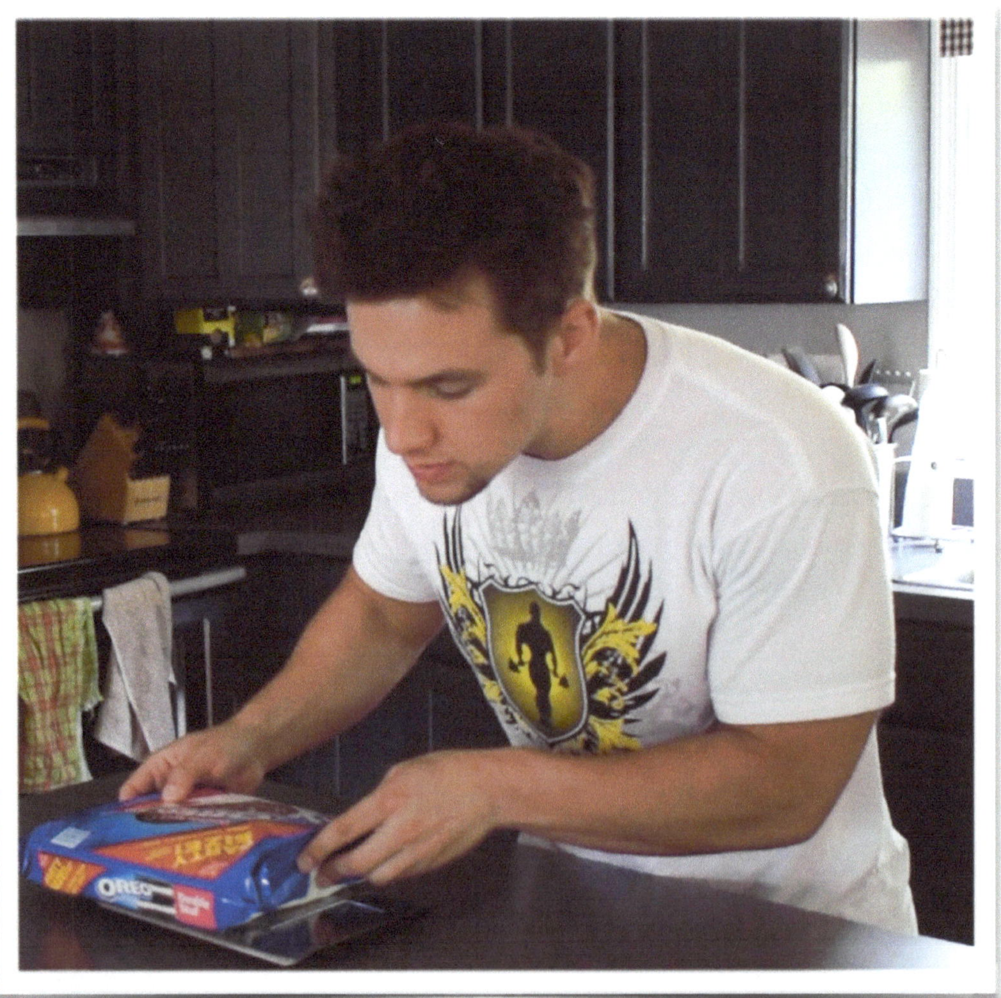

Even with your "treat" foods, accurate serving size is good to know.

METABOLISM

How It Works

Metabolism is basically defined as "the way things work in your body to keep you alive." That is a gross overestimation of what actually happens but it's the main point behind it. Our purpose is to demystify this word so that is no longer becomes the reason you may not be able to change your body.

While it is true that genetically, some people are simply born with a naturally higher or lower metabolic ability to utilize calories for energy, that isn't the end of the story. The good news is that your metabolism is in your power to manipulate. For the purpose of this book, we are going to look at ways to boost metabolism. That seems to be a common thread with the clients we have had over time and hopefully you'll feel better knowing that you are the one in control of your own health. At the end of this chapter, there will be some key points to take away to help boost your own metabolism but first, there are some things you need to know.

Fat Storage

The reason that our bodies store fat is that there is a surplus of energy. Our energy comes from the food we eat. It's just like putting gas in a car, except our version is in the form of carbohydrates, protein, and fat. Calories are the unit of energy that is stored in each of the macronutrients and every human body burns a given amount of them per day. Your body utilizes a specific number of calories to perform basic functions of survival such as heartbeat, brain activity, digestion, etc. This is called your "basal metabolic rate" or BMR. This number is determined by the size of your body and the energy it takes to maintain its composition as is.

Any activity you do above your BMR contributes to your "Total Daily Energy Expenditure" or TDEE. Think of it as simply BMR + Activity. This means that if your BMR was 1300 calories, and then throughout the day, you burned an additional 500 from exercise plus yet another additional 500 from regular activity such as playing with your children or climbing stairs, cleaning, playing sports, etc. that your TDEE would equal 2300. You could eat up to 2300 calories and store no fat for the day.

Eating more than that amount will cause your body to then store that excess energy (calories) for a later time when it is needed as fat. At the end of the day, fat loss and gain is that simple. This number is highly individualized and yes, genetics do play a role, but your body still needs to burn more calories in a day than it consumes.

Formula

"Formula? Nobody said anything about doing math!" I hear you say! Never fear, it is actually fairly simple. The first thing you need to keep in mind is that one pound of fat is worth about 3,500 calories on average. That is one pound of pure fat (at 9 calories per gram) and does not factor in how much water you are holding in or around those fat cells. But for the purposes of this book, we are aiming to keep things simple so let's only consider the loss of fat in our calorie goals and shedding excess water will be a bonus effect!

If we made a healthy realistic goal to lose one pound of fat per week, the deficit in calories would have to be 3,500 per week. Let's consider the previous example from the "Fat Storage" section of having a TDEE of 2300 calories per day. Multiply that by 7 days in a week and you would find that you burn 16,100 calories per week on average. This counts in BMR, exercise, and daily activity. In order to lose that one pound of fat, you would need to consume 3,500 less than the amount you burned. You would need to eat 12,600 calories for the week. Every day could potentially be different but by the end of the week, the energy balance would still need to be at the same deficit. The simplest way to calculate this in real life is to make this an even number of calories though, so divide by 7.

2,300 x 7 = 16,100 calories (burned) per week

16,100 − 3,500 = 12,600 calories per week

12,600 ÷ 7 = 1,800 calories per day

This fat loss formula can be applied in many different ways and if you wanted to lose more than a pound a week, you could increase the deficit. Proceed with great caution when going to extremes because the human body is nothing to toy with. We recommend making up this energy deficit in a safe way through small steps rather than simply through food deprivation alone. Our mission is to keep you healthy while feeling comfortable in your skin so try some of the following things to boost your TDEE:

- Go for multiple walks during the day
- Eat whole foods that take more energy to digest
- Park farther from the store in parking lots
- Take the stairs as opposed to the elevator
- If you work a desk job, stand up and move around every hour
- Work out in the morning as opposed to evening if possible
- Do workouts that incorporate more than one body part per day

TYPES OF DIETS

Before beginning this section, we should probably begin by defining what a diet is. To put it simply, a "diet" is just the way a person eats. The word should carry no extra connotation of health, time limit, etc. but due to clever marketing over the past few decades, it now comes with a lot of baggage. Our hope is that you will start to retrain your mind to only consider the word "diet" as a summary of the types of foods you eat.

It does seem that when relating to fitness and health, many people are continuously searching for the perfect diet —the one that will solve all of their woes and finally free them from the constant cycle of stress, adherence, and commitment issues. Before going too deep, we would like you to understand that there is no perfect diet, nor do we recommend following the latest trendy program simply because there are a smattering of people who are seeing results. The perfect diet is simply the one you can stick with for a long period of time. How do you envision yourself eating every day for the rest of your life?

Ketogenic

The ketogenic diet (or "keto" as it is commonly referred) has risen in popularity over the last few years due to the ease with which people can adhere to this form of eating. Similar to the Atkins diet that used to be popular, it is characterized by minimal amounts of carbohydrates, high fat, and moderate protein. There are a few differences in which the nutrient ratios differ but for the purposes of this, they function the same. The goal is to get the body to use fat as a primary energy source. The namesake of the diet comes from ketones being present in the bloodstream and used by the body and brain in place of carbohydrates for energy. These ketones are produced by the liver when fat is broken down.

The common macronutrient ratio for a ketogenic diet is 25% Protein, 5% Carbs, 70% Fat. These numbers are not rigid and different people will get different results. Some bodybuilders and athletes have reported protein percentages as high has around 40% of total caloric intake.

Pros	Cons
High fat foods can increase satiety	Favorite carb foods are eliminated
Even blood sugar levels through the day	Strength and endurance could decrease
Body doesn't retain excess water	Some micronutrients could become deficient

High Carb

A high carbohydrate diet is just what it sounds like—the majority of calories consumed are made up of carbohydrates. This type of diet is best suited for those who exert a high amount of energy during daily activity, such as athletes or individuals with a physically demanding job. As discussed in our Macros section, carbohydrates are the body's primary energy source. When performing vigorous activity such as working out, the body simply performs better when there is enough fuel to get the job done. Regardless of daily caloric surplus, deficit, or maintenance, the human body requires carbohydrates to function.

The macronutrient ratio for a high carb diet is really up to the individual but a tip for best absorption is to use a moderate to low amount of fat so that the carbohydrates digest effectively when needed.

*Almost by default, most plant-based diets are high carbohydrate.

Pros	Cons
Plenty of energy	Calories should be monitored based on goals
Food volume increases	Food volume increases
Variety of foods can help meet micronutrient needs better	Could lead to water retention if carb intake is too high

Low Carb

A common myth in the fitness world is that carbohydrates cause fat gain. This is not necessarily true. If a diet is exclusively carbohydrates (not recommended) and the total calories are not at a surplus, there will be no fat gain, simply because there is no extra energy to be stored.

A low carbohydrate diet typically has protein as the most abundant macronutrient by default, though a ketogenic diet is technically low carb as well. There is no defined macro ratio because once again, this is up to the individual. Our recommendation when considering a low carbohydrate approach is to use it sparingly or when you simply consumed too many carbohydrates the day before.

Pros	Cons
Can help remove excess water retention	Energy levels can drop
Easy way to restrict calories	Could cause low blood sugar
Can be used as a tool for aesthetic purposes	Mood may change

Low Fat

The low fat diet is a fad that began taking root in the health world in the early 1980's and persisted into the 2000's and only in the past decade or so has it finally begun to settle common popularity. The basic thinking was that "if you stop eating fat, you won't store fat," which is pretty far away from how fat storage actually works. Remember, fat is stored from excess calories overall, regardless of their source.

The standard marketing on low fat foods was predominantly around snack-type foods such as cookies, muffins, and even candy. The general replacement for the flavor fat would add to a food would be sugar, which coincidentally could lead to greater fat gain over time. It is our position that the weight lost by people during this time was more from an overall calorie deficit from removing more dense foods like eggs and meats from the diet as opposed to any correlation with fat intake specifically.

Pros	Cons
More room for carb intake	Missing vitamin profiles from fat sources
Possible easier digestion	Less satiety
Easy source of energy	Dietary fat aids in cellular health
	Blood sugar could fluctuate

Intermittent Fasting

Intermittent fasting is the most recent (as of this writing) dietary style in the health and fitness community. It is sometimes referred to as "time restricted eating" as well. Studies have been shown that fasting leads to increased bodily recovery, more stable dietary adherence, and even improved cellular health.

The most common approach is to use and 8 hour eating window with a 16 hour fasting window but the rules aren't that strict. Intermittent fasting is technically any time your stomach is empty and you aren't refilling it. We all fast when we sleep (hence "break-fast") and that is where the bulk of those hours come from in a more prolonged intermittent fast. Studies have proven that a fasting window of a minimum of 12 hours coordinates well with the brain and body's internal clock to begin receiving those fasting benefits. The actual time is completely up to the individual.

Pros	Cons
Could fight hunger	Could cause hunger
Improve metal clarity	Possible awkward social times (when fasting)
Larger, more satisfying meals	Could slow down metabolism

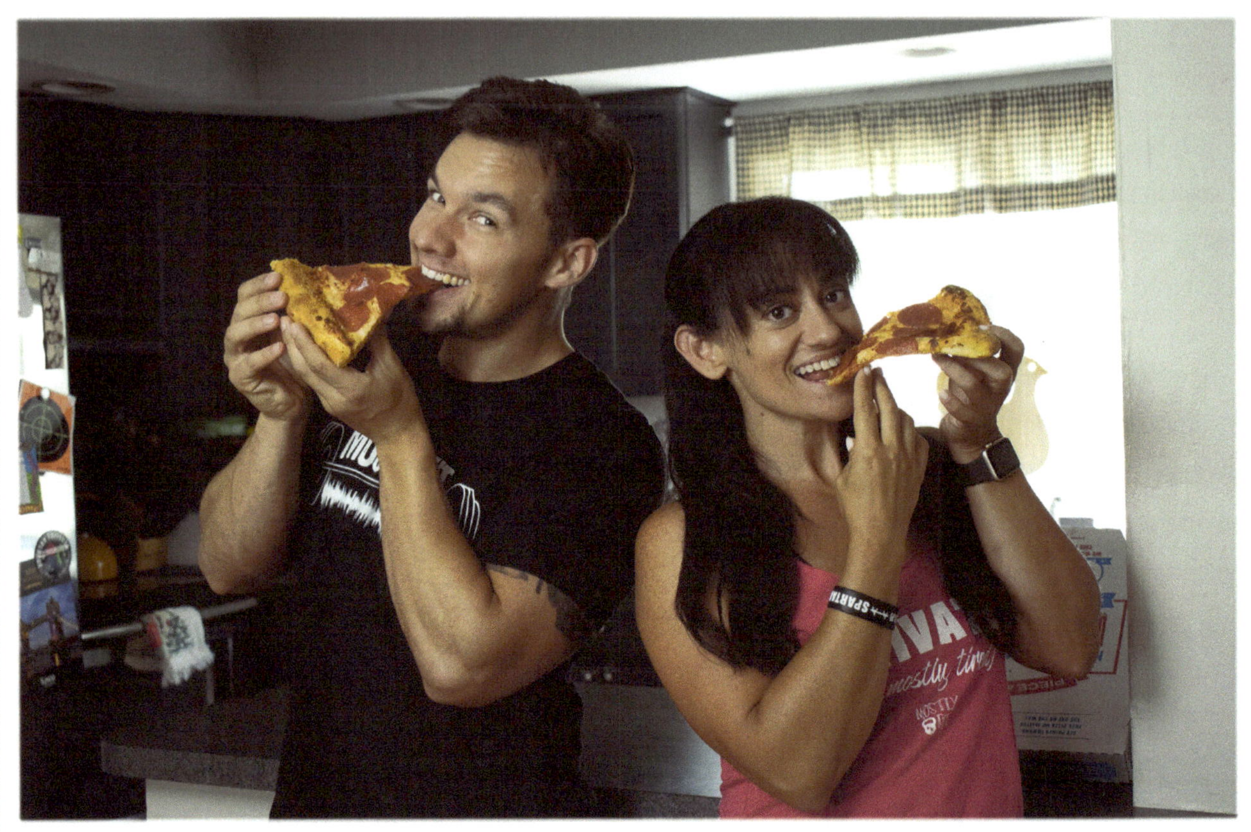

Pizza has carbs, fats, and a little bit of protein depending on the toppings.

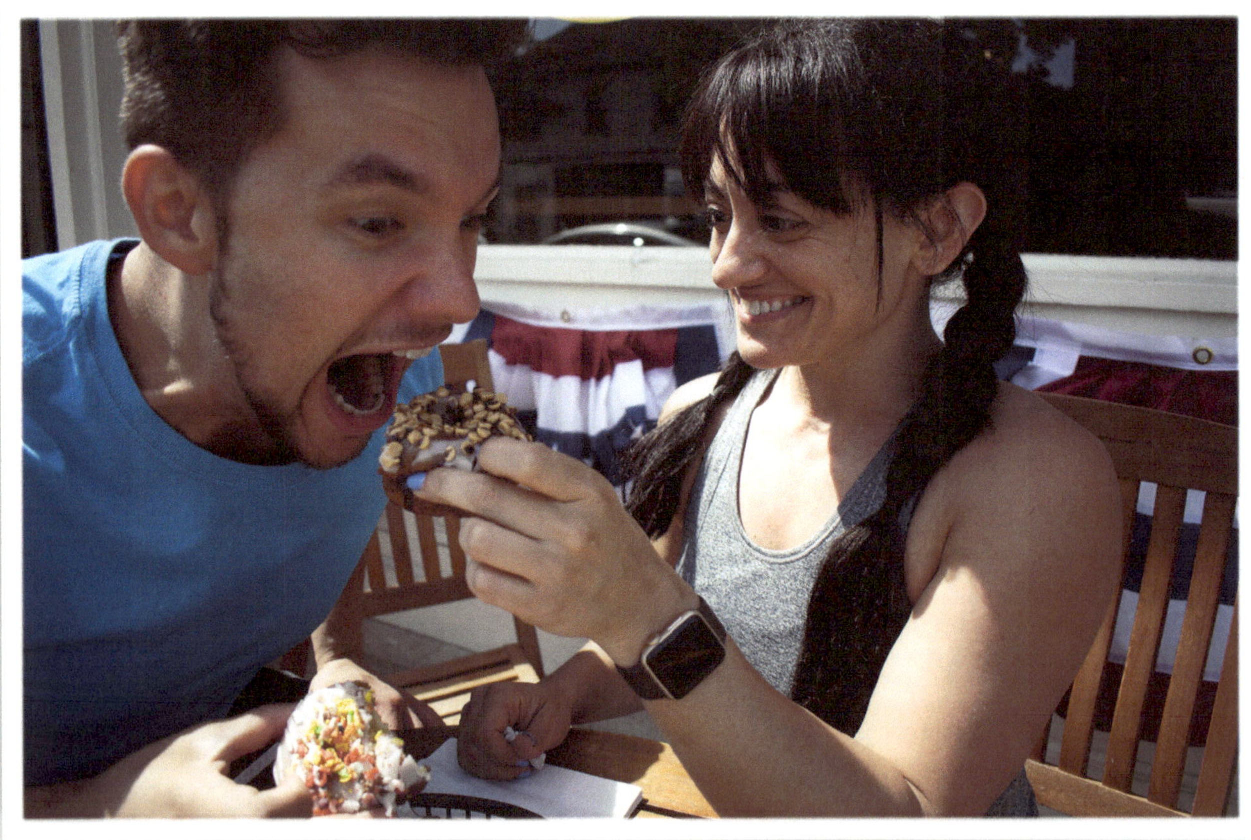

Too much sugar intake can lead to rapid fat storage. Be careful.

Carb Cycling

Carb cycling is way to basically keep the body guessing. Some people's metabolisms adjust very quickly and for this reason a little manipulation may be necessary. The goal with carb cycling is to maintain consistent protein and fat intake while only changing the amount of carbohydrates consumed. This will inherently change the caloric intake through the various stages of the cycle.

This process can be used for either aesthetic reasons to maintain an overall caloric deficit or for performance enhancement in which the higher carbohydrate intake will take place on days of more demanding activity such as distance running or various styles of strength training.

There are a few common ratios to easily implement carb cycling (low:high) 3:1, 2:1, 1:2, 5:2, or even a method of low, medium, high. The overall goal is to keep the body "guessing" to prevent fat gain or better aid in fat loss.

Pros	Cons
Unlikely to plateau	Constant focus on numbers
High carb days can be fun	Low carb days can be tough
Room for error	Room for error
Learning how food works	Lots to think about

Which One is Best?

Our approach is to build a diet around your goals and lifestyle. Looking forward to the foods you eat while having the energy to sustain your daily activities effectively is the way that we, as fitness professionals, choose to live. Sometimes things that don't fit any of these molds find their way into your day, and that's alright! That's the joy of living! Sometimes it's okay to have an extra glass of wine or dessert when it's not planned. No guilt should be associated with food in any way. We'll discuss more in the Metabolism section later!

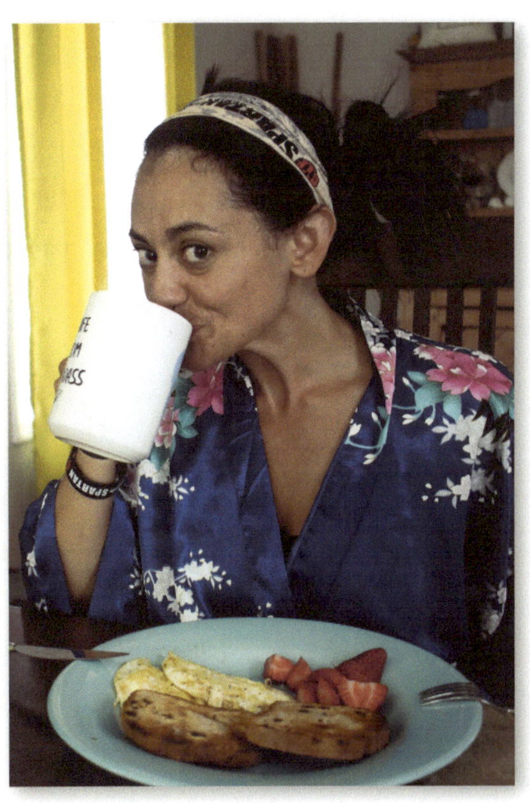

CHEATS

"So I get a cheat meal right?"

Cheat meals have been a source of controversy in the fitness world for as long as there has been a fitness world. In our modern world of social media, you can find on any given day someone with a lean athletic body indulging in some kind of delicious food that some might consider completely "off limits." There are some who have bragged about being able to have epic cheat days of 10,000 calories, some who have reported to be able to eat ice cream every night while losing tremendous amounts of fat, and yet others who see a cookie as the most wicked temptation. So what's the right answer?

Everyone is Different

The first fact that you should understand as you go through this guide is that every human being is different. Our genetic code is written differently, our minds are conditioned uniquely to our own experiences, and some peoples' bodies simply process nutrients differently. We even all have different cravings. A number of factors could be the cause of these cravings but we won't go into that here. What you need to know is that you will very likely have a vastly different relationship with food than the person next to you, both physiological and psychological. Therefore you must find your own path when it comes to what is considered "cheating on your diet." We would prefer you not even considering anything in that manner but it's a common phrase so we'll run with it. Hopefully we can help you decide the right path with the following information.

What is Cheating?

If we had to define "cheating" it would be classified as eating food that is outside of your defined dietary plan based on caloric and macronutrient needs. If your goal is to burn fat and build muscle and the same time, you would need to be at a caloric deficit for the day and meet a predetermined protein amount. If one day you haven't met that protein requirement and decide to just eat a chocolate cake for dinner, that would very likely be considered a cheat. However, should you beat yourself up for eating chocolate cake? Absolutely not!

When is it OK to Cheat?

For the sake of this example, let's say that you have a goal of losing one to two pounds a week, you've been following a consistent diet and workout regimen, going strong for the last month and lost your first nine pounds. Congratulations! You are on the right track and have been doing everything right! Now is probably a great time to allow yourself to indulge a little on some foods that aren't on your plan. If you want to go out for a night with the family, have an appetizer before a hearty dinner followed by dessert, you should enjoy it!

Now let's look at another common scenario. Say you just signed up with a personal trainer and started your new nutrition plan this past Monday. It's Friday and the past few days have felt like torture and you just need a break from that chicken, rice, and broccoli you've been eating every day at lunch. You're dying for something comfortable like a cookie! You've been sweating it out every day at the gym but may have not lost any weight yet. Maybe you did even lose a couple of pounds immediately. You deserve this right? Not so fast! If you haven't even gone one week without giving in to your old cravings, you probably want to take a step back and assess why you want those foods in the first place. Give it another week and try to incorporate more foods that you do enjoy into your meal plan so that you look forward to what you are eating on a daily basis. Then when something like a friend's birthday party comes around, you won't feel like you are being tempted with this wicked desire for a piece of cake but you can allow yourself to enjoy a reasonable amount without mentally going off the rails.

In short there is no defined time frame in which to have a cheat meal but should be based on your adherence to the plan you are following, your progress, and your mindset about the foods you are eating.

Cheat Days

In general, a healthy lifestyle shouldn't include full days of cheating. But there will inevitably come a time where you are on a family vacation or have a birthday weekend where you simply don't care about making healthy choices. You only get one shot at this life and you shouldn't feel guilty about enjoying those times. With that said though, you should definitely consider all of that in advance if you are attempting to change your body in any way. Just realize that on this occasion we are throwing caution to the wind and simply enjoying life. Once that is over, jump back on the routine you were on before and carry on! The worst that could happen is that you set yourself back a week in the grand scheme.

Full cheat days should not be a regular occurrence for general health, and if you are indeed in the process of transforming your body (and mind) they could keep you from making progress all together. Be warned.

THE BODY

We've spend a fair volume of this book on the nutrition aspect of fitness because that is generally the hardest part to get right when beginning a new lifestyle. It's also a struggle for those who have been involved for a while and have still heard all of the great rumors, myths, and marketing ploys and need to get back to basics. Now that we have that out of the way, it's time to talk about the reason health matters in the first place—your body. Once you know how to fuel it properly, you can begin to use it in the ways it was built to operate.

The human body is a wonderful and intricate design with agonist-antagonist relationships, self-healing tissues, automatic reflexes and as many other functions as you could imagine short of actual magic. When learning how to improve the movements of the body, it can be intimidating at first. Think of all the movements you may do throughout a single day! You may walk, move furniture, throw a ball, get out of the car, pull things from a high shelf, pick up a baby, you name it! Whether you're a teen athlete or a grandparent, knowing how your body functions is the first step in learning to make it function better.

Six Basic Moves

Going to the gym for the first time can be intimidating due to all of the machines, pulleys, bars, plates, etc. but instead of focusing on those, we would like for you to focus on the machine that is your body. How it works can control how all of those pieces of gym equipment work. There are some machines designed with a singular function in mind, but once you have mastered this simple knowledge, you will understand them so much better upon sight.

When broken down into the most basic of patterns, the human body moves in six different ways:

- Horizontal Pulling

- Horizontal Pushing

- Vertical Pulling

- Vertical Pushing

- Hip Dominant Leg Moves

- Knee Dominant Leg Moves

Every simple exercise will consist of one of these six movement patterns. This is admittedly an overly simplistic way to view strength but that is our entire focus after all. In our example workout plan later in the book, we will document how these movements apply to specific exercises, but for now, take a look at how they apply to real life and why you may want to strengthen that particular movement.

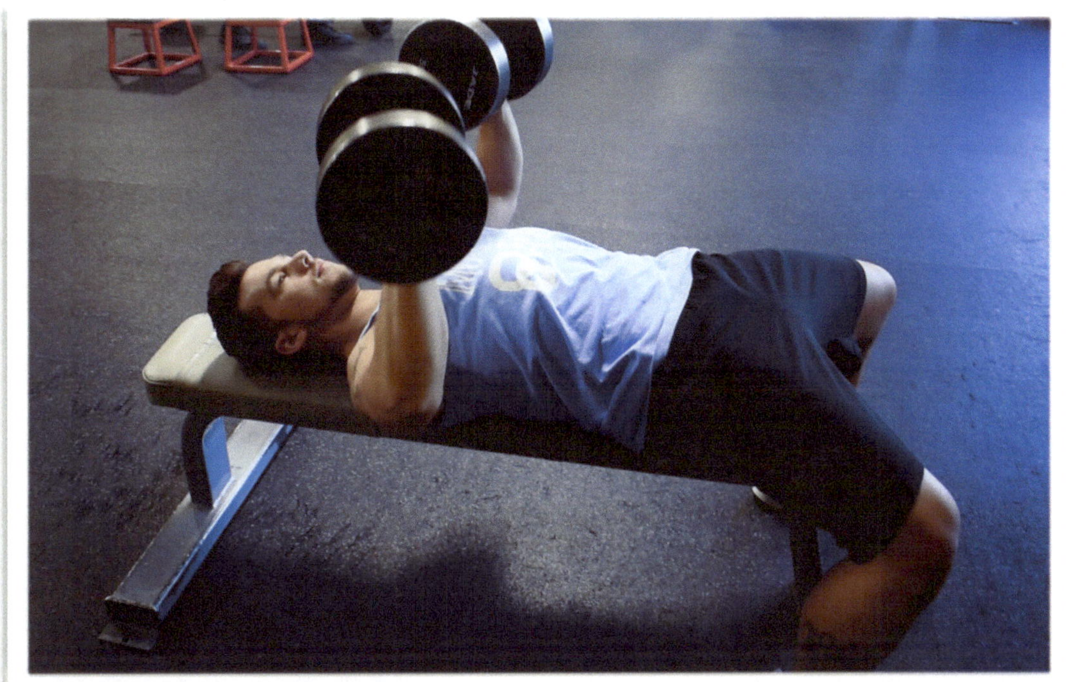

Count how many people do bench presses on Monday at the gym.

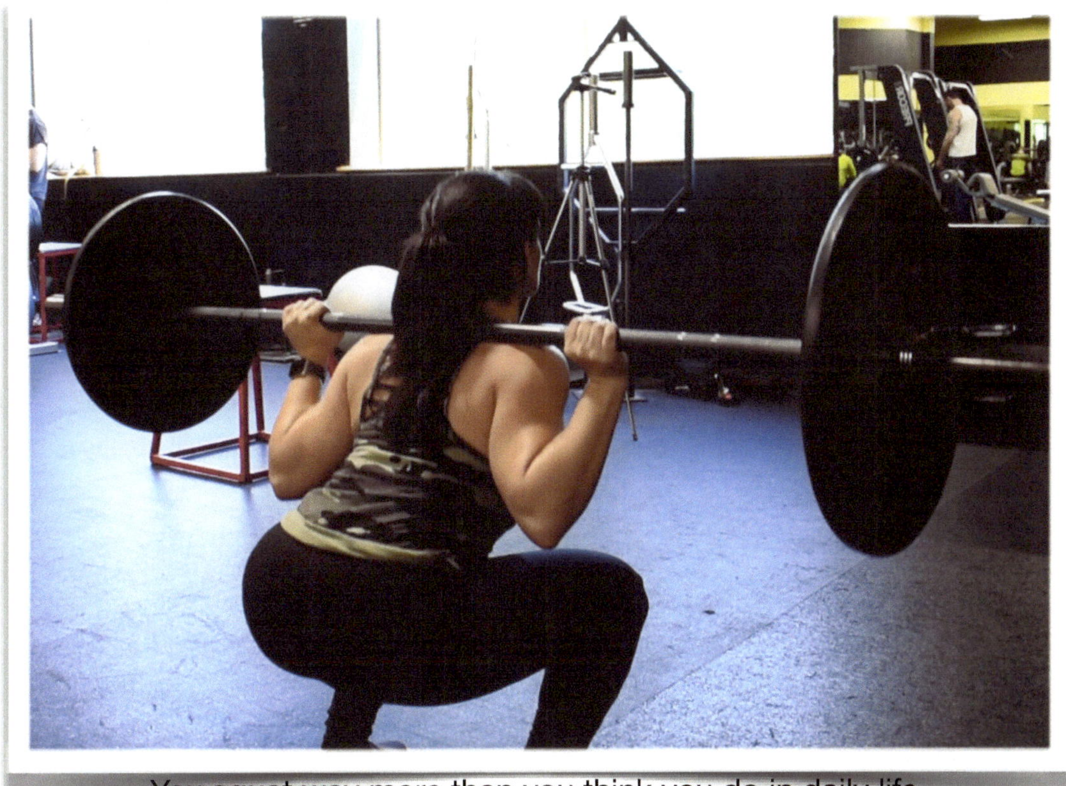

You squat way more than you think you do in daily life.

Parts of Strength

If your goal is more than just to make your body function better and your goal is more aesthetically based, you will want a little deeper knowledge in how muscles work specifically. These principles apply the way every muscle in your body works regardless of size or function.

Every muscle has an agonist (active) to antagonist (counteractive) relationship. Muscles can not push, they can only pull, so each muscle needs a muscles to work against it when it needs to let go of its tension. The easiest way to demonstrate this is the way your elbow bends. When you bend the elbow into "flexion" the biceps contract while the triceps relax. When you lower the elbow into "extension" the triceps contract while the biceps relax. This same function happens at each joint with its own group of muscles to control the movement. (This is one reason that we only rarely recommend splitting a program into body part days—balance is key).

Muscles themselves have three types of strength within them, all with different functions. These types of strength are:

- Concentric

- Eccentric

- Isometric

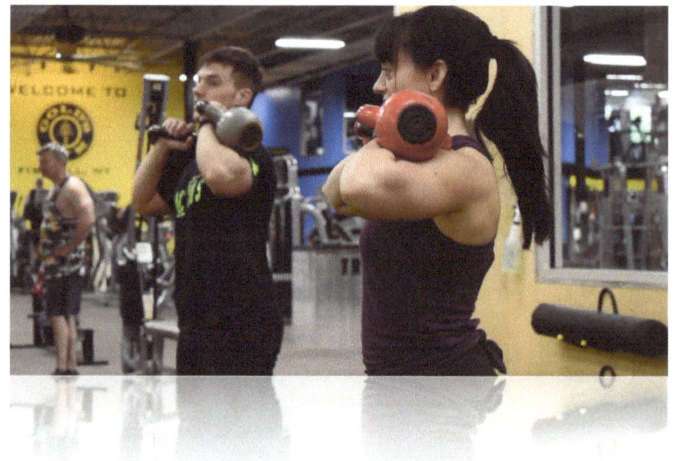

The concentric portion of the movement is when muscles contract and force is produced. This is not directly related to the way an object moves around the body, but the way the muscles function in order to create that movement.

The eccentric portion of the movement is commonly called the "negative." This is when the muscle is returning to a stretched position while still under tension. This part of strength allows you to maintain control while the negative is happening.

Isometric strength is a special type of strength because it holds things in place. When a muscle is contracted, maintaining that tension without movement is called an "isometric hold." There are special groups of muscle fibers that control all of these movements but we'll save that for a more advanced lesson.

Core Stability

"BUT WHAT ABOUT MY ABS?!" you're probably screaming at the book!

The core is arguably the most important part of physical fitness. It should be considered the foundation of all of your body's strength. Without core stability, the rest of your movements will greatly suffer and that leaves you at a higher risk for injury.

The abs are a special group of muscles that often don't get the type of love and attention for the job they do. The reason we saved those for this far into the chapter is simply because they are unique. The entire group of core musculature includes not only the abdominals but the obliques, glutes, spinal erectors, and a ton of internal muscles that perform the very important task of returning your spine to a safe neutral position and keeping it from getting too far out of line during movement. The function of your abs isn't to simply do crunches and sit-ups, but to prevent your spine from falling backward. They also have a relationship with muscles such as the spinal erectors and quadratus lumborum in the back, just like the biceps and triceps from before. Training the core for as much isometric stability as possible is one of the best approaches to core strength and function.

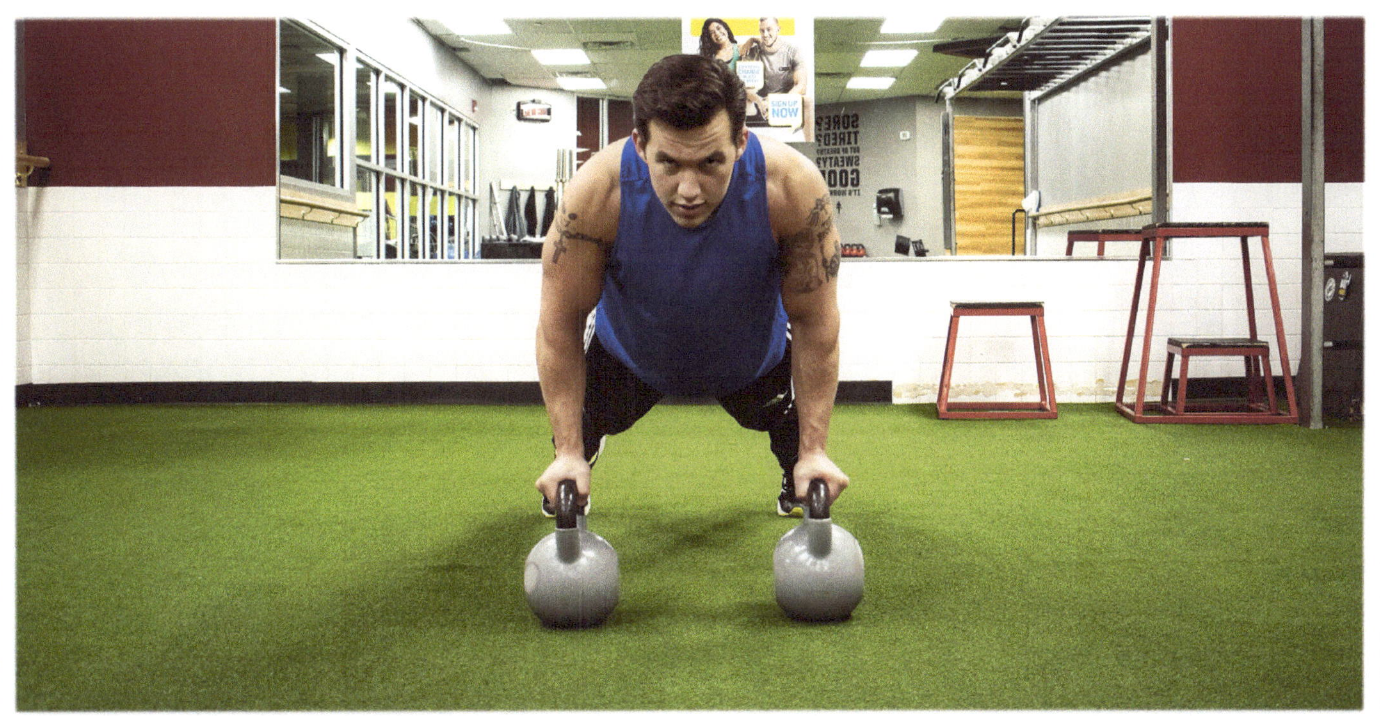

The group of muscles that form the core are designed to keep the spine neutral and safe.

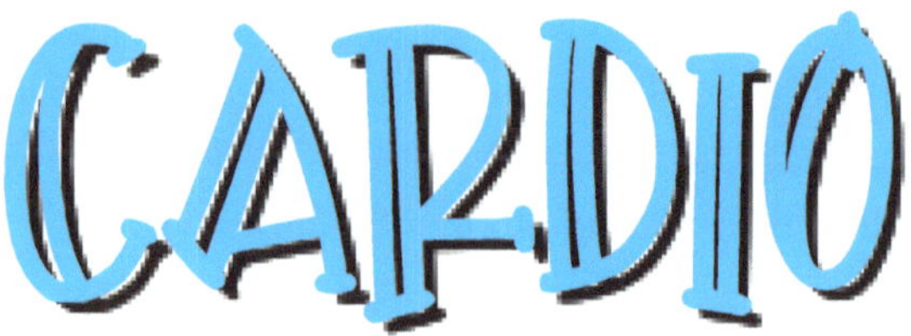

What Is It?

Cardio is simply a short term for "cardiovascular exercise." There is a pretty common consensus that cardio is one of the most boring activities in the gym, sometimes referred to as a "human hamster wheel." There are some gyms that are built around the amount of specifically cardio equipment they have, while other gyms like powerlifting gyms or hardcore dungeon style gyms that may have only one treadmill and bike in the entire place. This shows a little discrepancy in the perceived importance of cardiovascular activity does it not? Let's clear up the confusion!

Why You Need It

Cardiovascular exercises the most important muscle in the human body—your heart! The short answer to this is that, yes, you need some form of cardio in your life. The more efficient your heart is at pumping blood throughout your body, the better your nutrients can be dispersed and the better every single process in your body can function. Many studies have shown that cardiovascular disease is the leading cause of death in the world. The obvious antidote to that is to take care of your heart as much as you possibly can!

Annual Number of Deaths by Cause
(World) (2016)

Cause	Millions
Cardiovascular diseases	17.65
Cancers	8.93
Respiratory disease	3.54
Diabetes, blood and endocrine disease	3.19
Dementia	2.38
Lower respiratory infections	2.38
Neonatal deaths	1.73
Diarrheal diseases	1.66
Road incidents	1.34
Liver disease	1.26
Tuberculosis	1.21
Kidney disease	1.19
Digetive disease	1.09
HIV/AIDS	1.03
Suicide	0.81
Malaria	0.71
Homicide	0.39
Nutritional deficiencies	0.37
Meningitits	0.32
Protein-energy malnutrition	0.31
Drowning	0.23
Maternal deaths	0.21
Parkinson's disease	0.17
Alcohol disorder	0.16
Intestinal infectious diseases	0.14
Drug disorder	0.13
Hepatitis	0.13
Fire	0.13
Conflict	0.12
Heat-related deaths (hot or cold)	0.05
Terrorism	0.03
Natural disasters	0.01

https://en.wikipedia.org/wiki/List of causes of death by rate

"But what about fat loss?" you're probably screaming as you read this. Well, cardio does play a role in fat loss but it is not as big of a factor as many people believe. Doing cardio has indeed been shown to increase the calories burned for hours even after a workout is finished which means you will lose fat more efficiently. But there is more to the story.

The heart responds to the stimulus that is provided. If there is a demand for more blood flow to the various regions of the body, the heart rate begins to increase. The heart does not know whether you are on a treadmill, elliptical, mountainside, if there are kettlebells in your hands, or you are doing burpees. It only knows that more blood and oxygen is needed and for how long.

With that said, there are various types of cardio that you can do in or out of the gym to provide the required stimulus to the body in order to increase your heart rate over an extended period of time that will raise your metabolism, build endurance, and keep your heart healthy for a longer and more fulfilling life!

Steady State

Steady state cardio is the most common form of cardio that you will find in any gym. For this the heart is elevated significantly above its resting rate for an extended period of time anywhere from five minutes to an hour and beyond! There isn't much variation in this style of training and it is used for building endurance, burning additional calories, and recovery. You can also use it to catch up on some reading or your favorite TV shows (or our Youtube channel)!

Pros	Cons
Easy on the joints	Can get boring
Burn excess calories when needed	Too much can lead to muscle loss
Aids in post-workout recovery	Less time-efficient
Safe pre-workout warmup	Could deplete minerals from sweating
Can be performed every day	

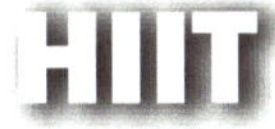 HIIT

High Intensity Interval Training, also known as HIIT, is another form of cardio exercise that has risen in popularity over the years. It is a more athletic style of training that can be used for a variety of purposes. In addition to a greater heart rate response, HIIT can be used to increase performance on a variety of movements such as running, jumping, and other creative things like burpees. The duration of activity is much shorter in the range of 15-45 seconds and incorporates intervals of rest for a short recovery in order to perform at maximum effort. The caveat to this is that the nervous system can't continue this kind of activity for as long as a typical steady state session until more advanced training stages. The recommended time is usually 8-10 minutes total and should not be done every day so as not to overexert the central nervous system.

Pros	Cons
Shorter duration	Taxing on the nervous system
Greater calorie burn per minute	Shorter intra-workout calorie burn
Long-lasting metabolic effect	Can be hindered by muscle imbalances
Boosts athletic performance and endurance	

Being Creative

The best approach to cardio, just like all other things, is a balanced one. We suggest taking this information and using pieces of it based on your goals to build a balanced program that incorporates a little of both worlds but not relying too heavily on either. Also, when doing HIIT training don't just rely on standard bodyweight movements, but try to add in things like kettlebells and timing the rests between your favorite weight lifting exercises. As previously stated, the heart doesn't know what caused the need for more blood flow and oxygen, just that it's needed.

In terms of body composition, the state of things on the inside will determine the way things look on the outside so if you haven't taken care of the dietary portion of your fitness journey, no amount of cardio is going to fix things. This is precisely the reason that the beginning majority of this guide is dedicated to the nutrition aspect of fitness. You must first have all the materials to build a house before you start swinging hammers.

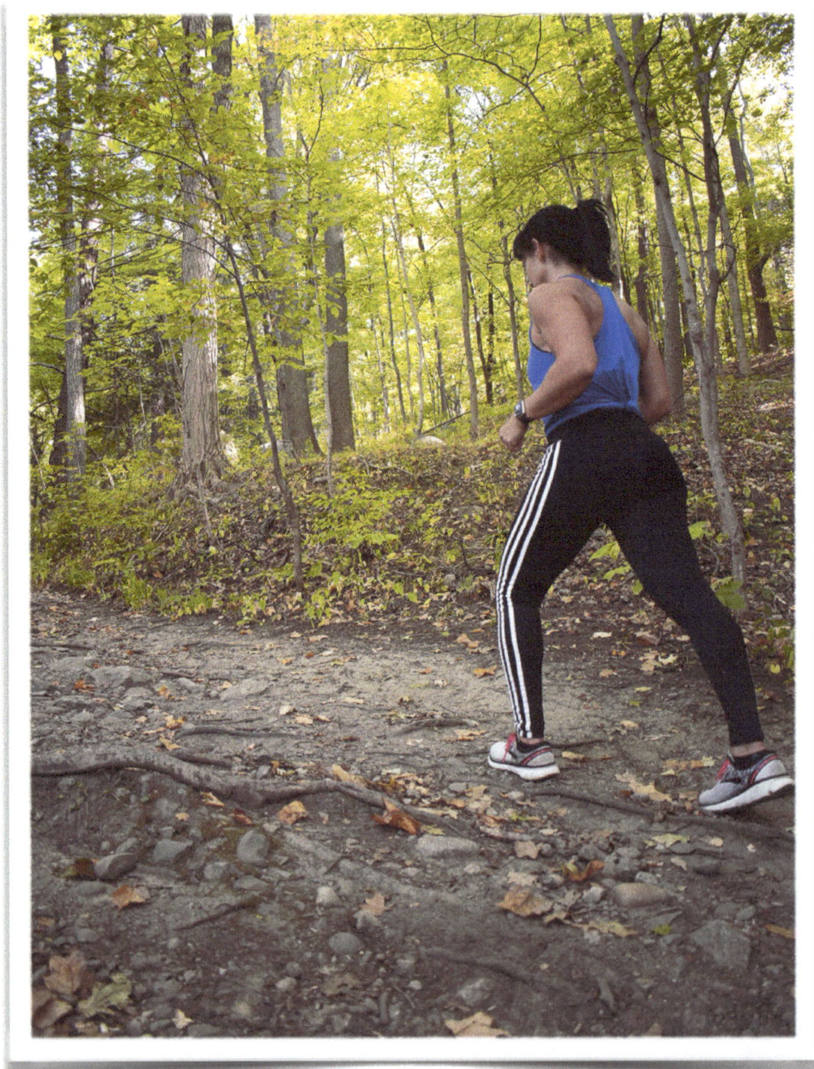

If you get bored, try cardio outside!

PLAN

Choosing Your Path

When you begin a workout routine, it is best to first think about the goal. Do you want to lose fat? Do you want to build muscle? Do you want to be able to accomplish a certain physical feat? All of these questions and more should determine the type of workout routine you choose. A healthy mix of strength and cardio will be the general guideline for most people but the way the program or even a single workout is structured would vary from a person whose goal is not the same as yours.

A person who is planning to run a marathon would do much more work in conditioning and strengthening all parts of the legs on top of the obvious running plan for cardiovascular conditioning. If the goal is to simply fit into an old pair of pants that won't button, we would recommend a full body weight training plan with minimal to moderate amounts of cardio. An aspiring bodybuilder may want to consider a higher volume in weight training and divide the body parts into different days.

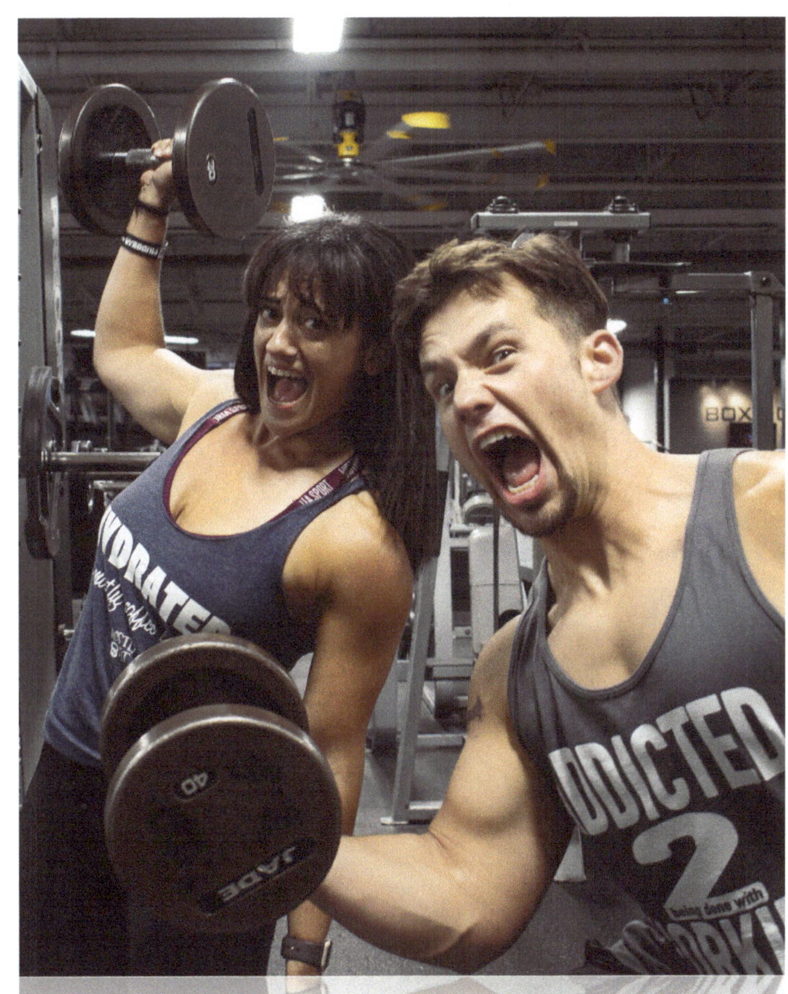

Every person is different so one workout does not fit all. In the next section we will provide you with a sample workout program to begin your own training regimen in a balanced way. If any of the exercises are questionable, please consult a fitness professional in your gym to prevent injury. Once you have mastered one workout routine in 30-90 days we recommend changing the routine to stimulate the body in a different way to always keep progressing physically (and mentally).

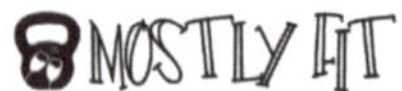

WORKOUTS

WARMUP

Exercise	Sets	Reps
Cardio	1	5 min
Prone Cobra	2	30s
Plank	2	30s
Side Plank	2	30s each
Glute Bridge	2	30s
Inchworm	2	5

***Warm Up Before Each Workout**

DAY 1

Exercise	Sets	Reps
Leg Press	3	10
DB Deadlift	3	10
Seated Row	3	10
Machine Bench Press	3	10
Cable Core Rotation	3	10e

DAY 2

Exercise	Sets	Reps
Goblet Squat to Bench	3	10
Barbell Row	3	10
Overhead DB Press	3	10
Wide Grip Lat Pulldown	3	10
Reverse Plank	3	30s

DAY 3

Exercise	Sets	Reps
Goblet Reverse Lunge	3	10
Cable Face Pull	3	10
DB Incline Bench Press	3	10
Reverse Grip Lat Pulldown	3	10
Russian Twist	3	30s

SAMPLE DAY OF EATING

This is a meal plan based on a person whose total daily energy expenditure is about 2500 calories and is trying to lose one pound of fat per week while maintaining strength and muscle size.

If this individual followed this meal plan exactly, it would have a nice variety of food types to maintain interest. It includes a little treat mid-afternoon with a protein bar to maintain satiety until dinner time. The variety in foods ensures a healthy balance of vitamins and minerals throughout the day as well. It also requires minimal amounts of preparation. It saves time but leaves out the guess work!

EXAMPLE

		Protein	Carbs	Fat
Total Calories	1948			
Macros (grams)		151	160	79
Breakfast	440	3 Eggs	3/4 cup Oats	(Egg Yolks)
Snack	248	Protein Shake	1/2 Banana	15 Almonds
Lunch	544	6oz Chicken Breast	Salad with Cranberries	Chopped Walnuts, Goat Cheese, Olive Oil
Snack	270	Clif Builder's Bar		
Dinner	388	5oz Ground Beef	1/2 cup Rice, 6 Brussel Sprouts	(Beef Fat)

THANK YOU

In Conclusion

We, Lindsay and Dizzy of Mostly Fit, would like to thank you for reading our first book. We realize that there is so much information out there in the fitness world due to marketing and mythology and it is important to have a basic foundation of knowledge to determine who to follow and what plan of action to take. The goal with this book has been to give you enough education to either get started or finally make everything click.

Ultimately, your fitness is in your hands because no personal trainer, motivational speech, or trendy supplement will get you to your goals unless you are willing to put in the work to make it happen. And when it comes to choosing that course of action, remember: the best routine is the one you will stick with. Don't pick a diet or workout plan that doesn't fit into your real life, but make sure to pick one! Try them all until you find something that sticks.

Once again, if you have any questions about the information in this guide, consult a fitness professional so that you will be safe. If you would like to contact us directly, we would be more than happy to help you out!

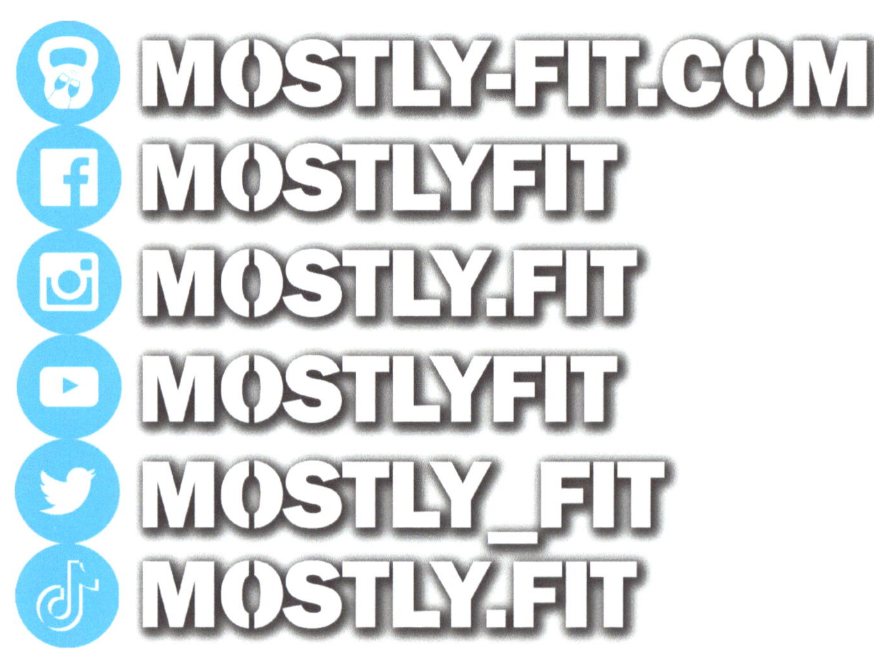

NOTES

NOTES

NOTES

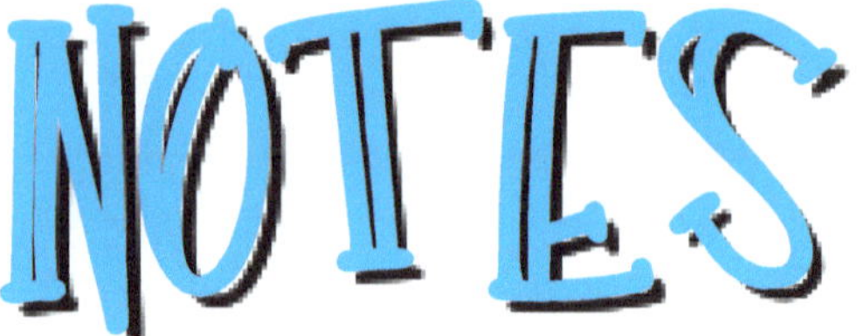

NOTES